The Complete Autoimmune Cookbook for Beginners

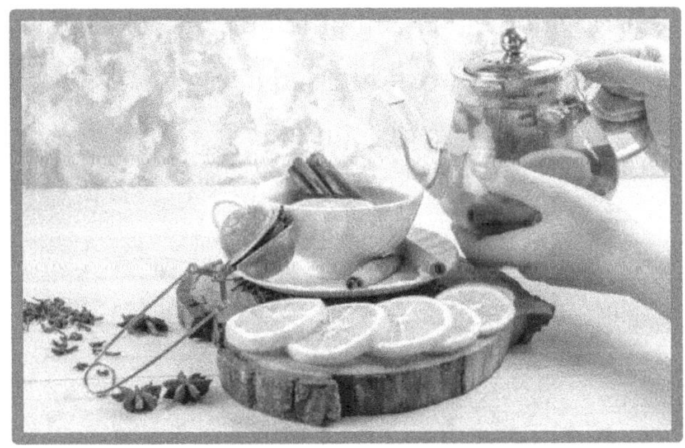

Nourishing your immune system with easy and delicious recipes

Janet Luck

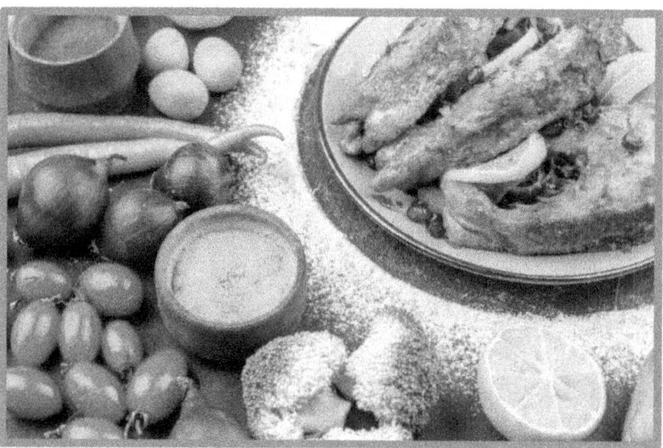

Disclaimer

The information provided in this book, "The Complete Autoimmune Cookbook for Beginners," is intended for educational purposes only and is not intended as a substitute for professional medical advice, diagnosis, or treatment. Always seek the advice of your physician or other qualified health provider with any questions you may have regarding a medical condition.

The author and publisher of this book are not responsible for any specific health or allergy needs that may require medical supervision and are not liable for any damages or negative consequences from any treatment, action, application, or preparation to any person reading or following the information in this book. References are provided for informational purposes only and do not constitute endorsement of any websites or other sources.

While the author has made every effort to ensure the accuracy and completeness of the information contained in this book, the author assumes no responsibility for errors, inaccuracies, omissions, or any inconsistency herein.

Contents

Introduction

Understanding Autoimmune Diseases

Autoimmune diseases are a group of disorders where the immune system, which typically defends the body against harmful invaders like bacteria and viruses, mistakenly attacks the body's own tissues. This abnormal response can affect various organs and systems, leading to a wide range of symptoms that can be chronic and debilitating.

The immune system's primary function is to distinguish between self and non-self. In autoimmune diseases, this distinction becomes blurred, causing the body to launch an immune response against its own cells. This self-attack can result in inflammation, tissue damage, and altered organ function. Over 80 different autoimmune diseases have been identified, each with its unique characteristics, though they often share common underlying mechanisms.

Some well-known autoimmune diseases include rheumatoid arthritis, where the immune system attacks the joints; multiple sclerosis, targeting the central nervous system; and type 1 diabetes, in which insulin-producing cells in the pancreas are destroyed. Other examples include lupus, which can affect multiple organs, and Hashimoto's thyroiditis, where the thyroid gland is the primary target.

The exact cause of autoimmune diseases remains unclear, but it is believed to involve a combination of genetic, environmental, and lifestyle factors. Genetic predisposition plays a significant role, as certain genes can make individuals more susceptible to developing autoimmune conditions. Environmental triggers such as infections, toxins, and stress are also thought to influence the onset and progression of these diseases. Additionally, hormonal changes, particularly in women, who are more commonly affected by autoimmune disorders, suggest a link to endocrine function.

Diagnosing autoimmune diseases can be challenging due to their diverse symptoms and overlap with other conditions. Blood tests to detect specific autoantibodies, imaging studies, and biopsies are commonly used to aid in diagnosis. Early and accurate diagnosis is crucial for managing symptoms and preventing irreversible damage.

Treatment for autoimmune diseases typically focuses on reducing inflammation, suppressing the immune response, and managing symptoms. This often involves the use of immunosuppressive medications, corticosteroids, and non-steroidal anti-inflammatory drugs (NSAIDs). In recent years, biologic therapies that target specific components of the immune system have become increasingly available, offering more precise treatment options.

Despite advances in medical treatments, many people with autoimmune diseases seek complementary approaches to improve their quality of life. Lifestyle modifications, including stress management, regular exercise, and adequate sleep, can play a significant role in managing symptoms. Additionally, diet has emerged as a crucial factor in supporting immune health and mitigating autoimmune responses.

The Role of Diet in Autoimmune Health

Diet plays a pivotal role in managing autoimmune diseases and supporting overall immune health. The food we consume can either exacerbate inflammation and autoimmune reactions or help to modulate the immune system and promote healing. Understanding the connection between diet and autoimmune health is essential for those living with these chronic conditions.

One of the primary dietary approaches for managing autoimmune diseases is the Autoimmune Protocol (AIP) diet. This elimination diet focuses on removing potential dietary triggers that may contribute to inflammation and autoimmune reactions. The AIP diet eliminates foods known to be common allergens or irritants, such as gluten, dairy, grains, legumes, nightshades, processed foods, and certain food additives. By removing these foods, individuals can reduce the burden on their immune system and allow the body to heal.

After a period of elimination, foods are gradually reintroduced one at a time to identify which foods may be causing symptoms. This process helps to create a personalized diet plan tailored to the individual's unique sensitivities and needs. Many people with autoimmune diseases find that the AIP diet helps to reduce symptoms, improve energy levels, and enhance overall well-being.

In addition to elimination diets like AIP, other dietary patterns have shown promise in supporting autoimmune health. The Mediterranean diet, rich in fruits, vegetables, whole grains, healthy fats, and lean proteins, has anti-inflammatory properties and is associated with a reduced risk of chronic diseases, including autoimmune conditions. The diet's emphasis on omega-3 fatty acids from fish, nuts, and seeds helps to modulate the immune response and reduce inflammation.

Another important aspect of diet in autoimmune health is gut health. The gut plays a central role in the immune system, housing a significant portion of immune cells and influencing immune function. A healthy gut microbiome, the community of beneficial bacteria in the digestive tract, is crucial for maintaining immune balance and preventing autoimmune reactions. Consuming probiotic-rich foods like yogurt, kefir, sauerkraut, and fermented vegetables can help to support a healthy gut microbiome. Additionally, prebiotic foods such as garlic, onions, leeks, and asparagus provide nourishment for beneficial bacteria, promoting gut health and immune function.

Nutrient-dense foods are essential for supporting immune health and managing autoimmune diseases. Vitamins and minerals like vitamin D, vitamin A, vitamin C, zinc, and selenium play critical roles in immune function and inflammation regulation. Ensuring adequate intake of these nutrients through a varied and balanced diet is important for individuals with autoimmune conditions.

While diet is a powerful tool for managing autoimmune diseases, it is important to approach dietary changes with guidance from healthcare professionals. Each person's experience with autoimmune disease is unique, and what works for one individual may not work for another. A registered dietitian or nutritionist with experience in autoimmune conditions can provide personalized recommendations and support for dietary changes.

How to Use This Cookbook

"The Complete Autoimmune Cookbook for Beginners" is designed to be a practical and comprehensive guide for individuals seeking to manage their autoimmune conditions through diet. This cookbook offers a variety of recipes, meal planning tips, and educational resources to help you navigate the complexities of autoimmune health and enjoy delicious, nourishing meals.

To get the most out of this cookbook, it is important to understand its structure and how to use it effectively. The book is divided into several chapters, each focusing on different aspects of the autoimmune protocol (AIP) diet and providing recipes tailored to support autoimmune health.

Start with the introductory chapters, which provide essential information about autoimmune diseases and the role of diet in managing these conditions. These chapters will help you understand the basics of the AIP diet, the foods to avoid, and the foods to include. You'll also find tips for transitioning to an AIP diet and essential kitchen tools that will make meal preparation easier.

The meal planning and preparation chapter offers practical advice on how to plan your meals, shop for groceries, and prepare food in advance. This section includes a sample 7-day meal plan to help you get started and a list of pantry staples that are essential for an AIP diet. Planning and preparation are key to successfully following the AIP diet, and this chapter will provide you with the tools and strategies you need to stay on track.

The recipe chapters are organized by meal type, including breakfast, lunch, dinner, snacks, appetizers, and desserts. Each recipe is designed to be simple, flavorful, and compliant with the AIP diet. You'll find a variety of dishes to suit different tastes and preferences, ensuring that you can enjoy a diverse and satisfying diet while managing your autoimmune condition.

Each recipe includes clear instructions, ingredient lists, and nutritional information to help you make informed choices. Many recipes also offer tips for substitutions and modifications, allowing you to adapt the dishes to your specific needs and preferences. Whether you're looking for a quick and easy breakfast, a hearty dinner, or a sweet treat, this cookbook has something for everyone.

Throughout the book, you'll find helpful tips and insights to support your journey on the AIP diet. From batch cooking and meal prep strategies to ideas for incorporating more nutrient-dense foods into your diet, these tips are designed to make the AIP diet more manageable and enjoyable.

Remember, the goal of this cookbook is not only to provide you with delicious recipes but also to empower you with knowledge and skills to take control of your health. By following the AIP diet and incorporating the recipes and tips in this book, you can reduce inflammation, manage your symptoms, and improve your overall well-being.

While this cookbook is a valuable resource, it is important to consult with your healthcare provider before making any significant dietary changes, especially if you have specific medical conditions or concerns. A registered dietitian or nutritionist with experience in autoimmune conditions can provide personalized guidance and support to help you achieve your health goals.

We hope that "The Complete Autoimmune Cookbook for Beginners" becomes a trusted companion on your journey to better health. Enjoy exploring the recipes, experimenting with new ingredients, and discovering the many delicious ways to nourish your body while managing your autoimmune condition.

Chapter 1: Breakfast Recipes

Energizing Smoothies and Juices

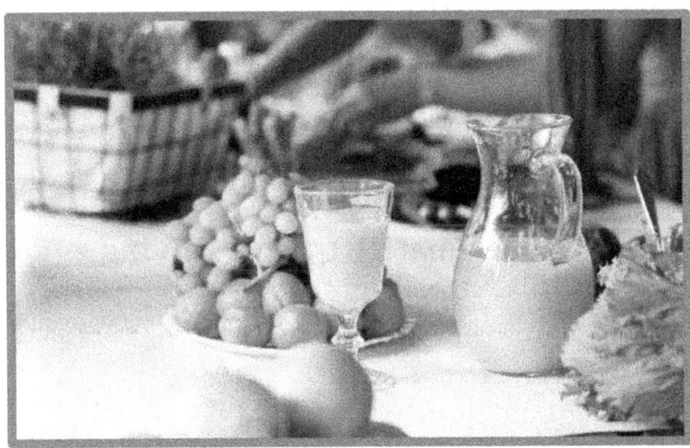

Smoothies and juices can be a quick and nutritious way to start your day, providing essential vitamins and minerals while being easy on the digestive system. Here are a few AIP-friendly recipes to energize your mornings.

1. Green Detox Smoothie

Ingredients:

- 1 cup spinach

- 1/2 cucumber

- 1 green apple, cored and sliced

- 1/2 avocado

- 1 cup coconut water

- 1 tablespoon fresh lemon juice

Preparation Method:

- Add all ingredients to a blender.

- Blend until smooth.

- Serve immediately.

Calories: Approximately 150 per serving

2. Berry Bliss Smoothie

Ingredients:

- 1 cup mixed berries (strawberries, blueberries, raspberries)

- 1/2 banana

- 1 cup coconut milk

- 1 tablespoon collagen peptides (optional for extra protein)

- 1 teaspoon honey (optional)

Preparation Method:

- Combine all ingredients in a blender.

- Blend until creamy and smooth.
- Pour into a glass and enjoy.

Calories: Approximately 200 per serving

3. Carrot-Orange Juice

Ingredients:

- 3 large carrots, peeled
- 2 oranges, peeled
- 1-inch piece of ginger, peeled

Preparation Method:

- Pass all ingredients through a juicer.
- Stir well and serve over ice if desired.

Calories: Approximately 120 per serving

Grain-Free Pancakes and Waffles

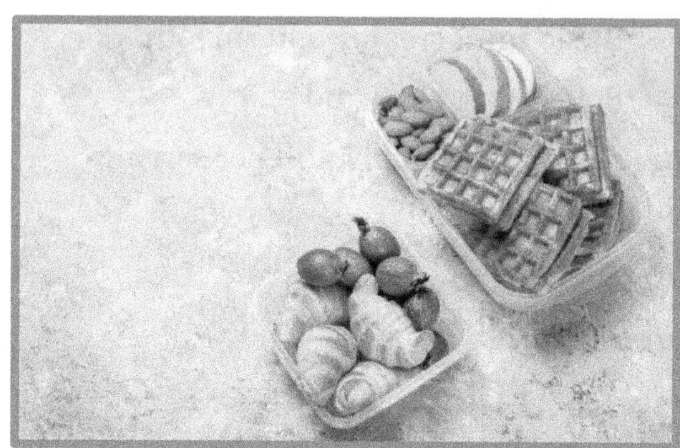

Grain-free pancakes and waffles are a delicious way to enjoy a classic breakfast favorite while staying compliant with the AIP diet.

1. Cassava Flour Pancakes

Ingredients:

- 1 cup cassava flour
- 1 cup coconut milk
- 2 tablespoons olive oil
- 1 tablespoon honey
- 1/2 teaspoon baking soda
- Pinch of salt

Preparation Method:

- In a bowl, combine all ingredients and mix until smooth.
- Heat a skillet over medium heat and lightly grease with olive oil.
- Pour 1/4 cup of batter onto the skillet and cook until bubbles form.
- Flip and cook until golden brown.
- Serve with fresh fruit or maple syrup.

Calories: Approximately 90 per pancake

2. Sweet Potato Waffles

Ingredients:

- 1 cup cooked and mashed sweet potatoes
- 1/2 cup coconut flour
- 1/2 cup coconut milk
- 1/4 cup olive oil
- 1 tablespoon honey
- 1/2 teaspoon baking soda
- Pinch of salt

Preparation Method:

- Preheat the waffle iron and lightly grease with olive oil.

- In a bowl, mix all ingredients until well combined.
- Pour batter into the waffle iron and cook according to manufacturer's instructions.
- Serve with coconut yogurt or fresh fruit.

Calories: Approximately 150 per waffle

Egg-Free Scrambles and Hashes

Egg-free scrambles and hashes can provide a hearty and satisfying breakfast without the need for eggs, making them perfect for the AIP diet.

1. Butternut Squash and Kale Hash

Ingredients:
- 1 small butternut squash, peeled and cubed
- 1 cup kale, chopped
- 1/2 onion, diced
- 1 tablespoon olive oil
- 1/2 teaspoon turmeric

- Salt and pepper to taste

Preparation Method:

- Heat olive oil in a skillet over medium heat.
- Add onion and cook until translucent.
- Add butternut squash and cook until tender.
- Stir in kale and turmeric, cooking until kale is wilted.
- Season with salt and pepper and serve.

Calories: Approximately 180 per serving

2. Mushroom and Spinach Scramble

Ingredients:

- 1 cup mushrooms, sliced
- 1 cup spinach
- 1/2 zucchini, diced
- 1 tablespoon olive oil
- 1/2 teaspoon garlic powder
- Salt and pepper to taste

Preparation Method:

- Heat olive oil in a skillet over medium heat.
- Add mushrooms and zucchini, cooking until soft.

- Stir in spinach and garlic powder, cooking until spinach is wilted.
- Season with salt and pepper and serve.

Calories: Approximately 130 per serving

3. Sweet Potato and Apple Hash

Ingredients:

- 1 large sweet potato, peeled and cubed
- 1 apple, cored and diced
- 1/2 onion, diced
- 1 tablespoon coconut oil
- 1/2 teaspoon cinnamon
- Salt to taste

Preparation Method:

- Heat coconut oil in a skillet over medium heat.
- Add onion and cook until soft.
- Add sweet potato and cook until tender.
- Stir in apple and cinnamon, cooking until apple is soft.
- Season with salt and serve.

Calories: Approximately 210 per serving

These recipes provide a variety of nutritious and delicious options to start your day, ensuring you get the energy and nutrients needed while following the AIP diet.

Nut-Free Granolas and Porridges

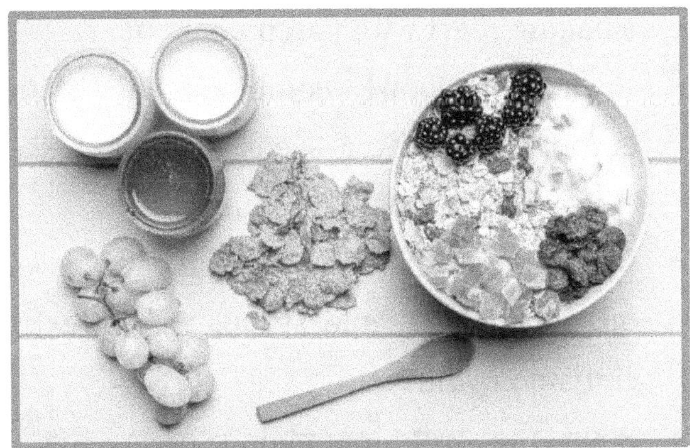

1. Coconut Crunch Granola

Ingredients:

- 2 cups shredded coconut
- 1 cup sunflower seeds
- 1 cup pumpkin seeds

- 1/2 cup chia seeds
- 1/2 cup dried cranberries (unsweetened)
- 1/4 cup coconut oil, melted
- 1/4 cup honey or maple syrup
- 1 teaspoon vanilla extract
- 1/2 teaspoon cinnamon
- Pinch of salt

Preparation Method:

- Preheat your oven to 300°F (150°C) and line a baking sheet with parchment paper.
- In a large bowl, combine the shredded coconut, sunflower seeds, pumpkin seeds, chia seeds, and dried cranberries.
- In a separate bowl, mix the melted coconut oil, honey or maple syrup, vanilla extract, cinnamon, and salt.
- Pour the wet ingredients over the dry ingredients and mix well until everything is evenly coated.
- Spread the mixture evenly on the prepared baking sheet.

- Bake for 20-25 minutes, stirring halfway through, until the granola is golden brown and crispy.
- Allow the granola to cool completely before storing it in an airtight container.

Calories: Approximately 200 calories per 1/2 cup serving.

2. Seed and Fruit Granola

Ingredients:

- 1 cup rolled oats (gluten-free if necessary)
- 1/2 cup sunflower seeds
- 1/2 cup pumpkin seeds
- 1/2 cup dried apricots, chopped
- 1/4 cup flaxseeds
- 1/4 cup coconut oil, melted
- 1/4 cup maple syrup
- 1 teaspoon cinnamon
- Pinch of salt

Preparation Method:

- Preheat the oven to 300°F (150°C) and line a baking sheet with parchment paper.

- In a large bowl, mix together the rolled oats, sunflower seeds, pumpkin seeds, dried apricots, and flaxseeds.
- In another bowl, whisk together the melted coconut oil, maple syrup, cinnamon, and salt.
- Pour the wet ingredients over the dry mixture and stir until well combined.
- Spread the granola mixture evenly on the baking sheet.
- Bake for 25-30 minutes, stirring halfway through, until the granola is golden and fragrant.
- Let the granola cool completely before storing it in an airtight container.

Calories: Approximately 180 calories per 1/2 cup serving.

Nut-Free Porridge Recipes

1. Coconut Quinoa Porridge

Ingredients:

- 1 cup quinoa, rinsed

- 1 can (14 oz) coconut milk

- 1 cup water

- 2 tablespoons honey or maple syrup

- 1 teaspoon vanilla extract

- 1/2 teaspoon cinnamon

- Fresh fruit for topping (e.g., berries, bananas)

Preparation Method:

- In a medium saucepan, combine the quinoa, coconut milk, and water. Bring to a boil.

- Reduce heat to low, cover, and simmer for about 15 minutes, or until the quinoa is tender and the liquid is absorbed.

- Stir in the honey or maple syrup, vanilla extract, and cinnamon.

- Serve warm, topped with fresh fruit.

Calories: Approximately 250 calories per serving.

2. Apple Cinnamon Amaranth Porridge

Ingredients:

- 1 cup amaranth

- 2 cups water
- 1 apple, peeled and diced
- 1 teaspoon cinnamon
- 1 tablespoon honey or maple syrup
- 1/4 cup raisins
- 1/4 cup coconut milk

Preparation Method:

- Combine the amaranth and water in a medium saucepan. Bring to a boil.
- Reduce heat to low, cover, and simmer for about 20 minutes, stirring occasionally, until the amaranth is tender.
- Stir in the diced apple, cinnamon, honey or maple syrup, raisins, and coconut milk.
- Cook for an additional 5 minutes, until the apples are tender and the porridge is creamy.
- Serve warm.

  Calories: Approximately 220 calories per serving.

Healing Teas and Elixirs

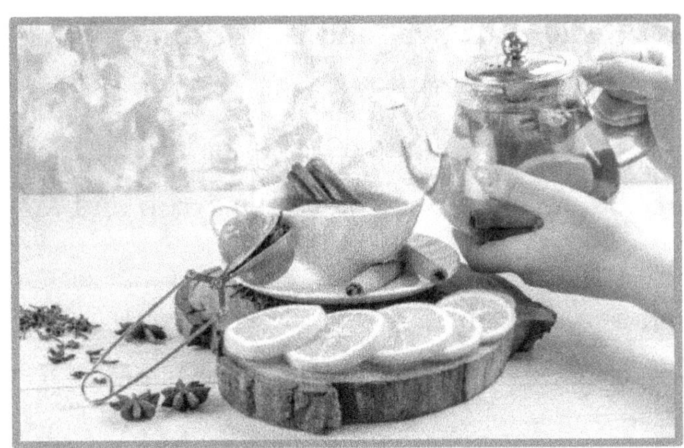

Healing Tea Recipes

1. Ginger Turmeric Tea

Ingredients:

- 1-inch piece of fresh ginger, sliced
- 1-inch piece of fresh turmeric, sliced
- 1 tablespoon honey or maple syrup
- Juice of 1 lemon
- 4 cups water

Preparation Method:

- In a medium saucepan, bring the water to a boil.
- Add the sliced ginger and turmeric.

- Reduce the heat and let it simmer for 10-15 minutes.
- Strain the tea into a teapot or large jar.
- Stir in the honey or maple syrup and lemon juice.
- Serve warm.

Calories: Approximately 25 calories per cup.

2. Peppermint Chamomile Tea

Ingredients:

- 1 tablespoon dried peppermint leaves
- 1 tablespoon dried chamomile flowers
- 4 cups water
- 1 tablespoon honey or maple syrup (optional)

Preparation Method:

- Bring the water to a boil in a medium saucepan.
- Remove from heat and add the dried peppermint and chamomile.
- Cover and let steep for 10 minutes.
- Strain the tea into a teapot or large jar.
- Stir in honey or maple syrup if desired.

6. Serve warm or chilled.

Calories: Approximately 20 calories per cup (with honey).

1. Golden Milk Elixir

- **Ingredients**:
  - 2 cups coconut milk
  - 1 teaspoon turmeric powder
  - 1/2 teaspoon cinnamon
  - 1/4 teaspoon black pepper
  - 1 tablespoon honey or maple syrup
  - 1/2 teaspoon vanilla extract

Preparation Method:

- In a small saucepan, combine the coconut milk, turmeric, cinnamon, and black pepper.
- Heat over medium heat, stirring frequently, until warm but not boiling.
- Remove from heat and stir in the honey or maple syrup and vanilla extract.
- Pour into mugs and serve warm.

Calories: Approximately 180 calories per cup.

2. Lemon Ginger Detox Elixir

Ingredients:

- 4 cups water
- 1-inch piece of fresh ginger, sliced
- Juice of 2 lemons
- 1 tablespoon apple cider vinegar
- 1 tablespoon honey or maple syrup

Preparation Method:

- In a medium saucepan, bring the water and sliced ginger to a boil.
- Reduce heat and let it simmer for 10 minutes.
- Strain the ginger out and pour the liquid into a pitcher.
- Stir in the lemon juice, apple cider vinegar, and honey or maple syrup.
- Serve warm or chilled.

Calories: Approximately 30 calories per cup.

These recipes provide a variety of options for creating nut-free granolas and porridges as well as healing teas and elixirs that are both delicious and beneficial for your health. Each recipe is designed to support an anti-inflammatory diet, providing nourishing and comforting foods and beverages to help manage autoimmune conditions.

Chapter 2: Lunch Recipes

Nourishing Soups and Stews

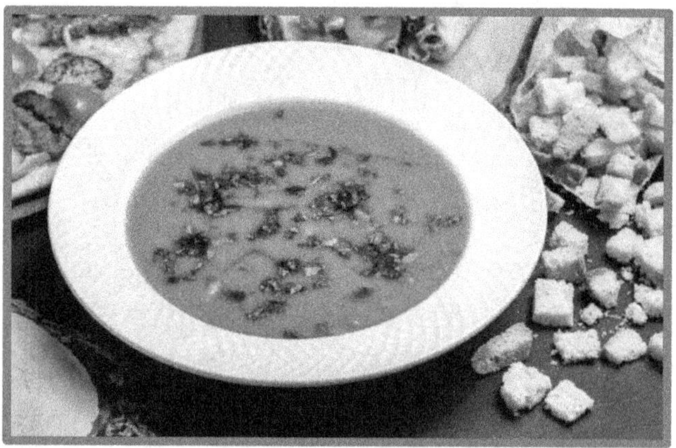

1. Chicken and Vegetable Soup

Ingredients:

- 2 chicken breasts (300g), diced
- 2 carrots, diced
- 2 celery stalks, diced
- 1 onion, diced
- 2 cloves garlic, minced
- 1 zucchini, diced
- 4 cups chicken broth
- 1 tsp thyme

- Salt and pepper to taste

Preparation Method:

- In a large pot, heat a small amount of oil over medium heat. Add diced chicken and cook until browned.
- Add garlic and onion, sauté until softened.
- Add carrots, celery, and zucchini. Cook for 5 minutes.
- Pour in the chicken broth and add thyme, salt, and pepper.
- Bring to a boil, then reduce heat and simmer for 20 minutes.

<u>Calories:</u> 250 per serving

2. Beef and Sweet Potato Stew

Ingredients:

- 1 lb beef stew meat, cubed
- 2 sweet potatoes, peeled and cubed
- 1 onion, chopped
- 2 cloves garlic, minced
- 1 cup beef broth
- 1 cup water

- 1 tsp rosemary
- Salt and pepper to taste

Preparation Method:

- Brown the beef in a large pot over medium heat.
- Add garlic and onion, sauté until fragrant.
- Add sweet potatoes, beef broth, water, rosemary, salt, and pepper.
- Bring to a boil, reduce heat, and simmer for 1 hour.

Calories: 320 per serving

Lunch Recipes: Satisfying Sandwich Alternatives

1. Collard Green Wraps with Turkey and Avocado

Ingredients:

- 4 large collard green leaves
- 8 slices turkey breast
- 1 avocado, sliced

- 1 tomato, sliced

- 1 cucumber, sliced

- 1 tbsp Dijon mustard

Preparation Method:

- Spread mustard on each collard green leaf.

- Layer with turkey, avocado, tomato, and cucumber.

- Roll tightly, securing with toothpicks if necessary.

Calories: 200 per wrap

2. Portobello Mushroom Burger

Ingredients:

- 2 large portobello mushrooms

- 4 oz ground turkey

- 1 slice tomato

- 1 slice red onion

- Lettuce leaves

- 1 tsp olive oil

Preparation Method:

- Preheat oven to 375°F (190°C).

- Brush mushrooms with olive oil and bake for 15 minutes.
- Grill the turkey patty until cooked through.
- Assemble with turkey patty, tomato, onion, and lettuce between two mushroom caps.

Calories: 350 per burger

Lunch Recipes: Hearty and Healthy Bowlsqqq

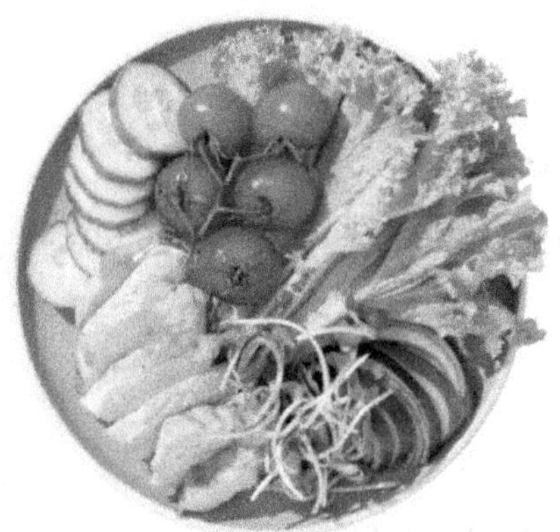

1. Quinoa and Roasted Veggie Bowl

Ingredients:

- 1 cup quinoa, cooked

- 1 cup roasted vegetables (zucchini, bell peppers, carrots)
- 1/2 cup chickpeas, drained and rinsed
- 2 tbsp tahini dressing

Preparation Method:

- Cook quinoa according to package instructions.
- Roast vegetables in the oven at 400°F (200°C) for 25 minutes.
- Assemble the bowl with quinoa, roasted veggies, chickpeas, and drizzle with tahini dressing.

Calories: 450 per bowl

2. Teriyaki Chicken Bowl

Ingredients:

- 1 chicken breast (150g), sliced
- 1 cup broccoli florets
- 1/2 cup carrots, julienned
- 1 cup brown rice, cooked
- 2 tbsp teriyaki sauce

Preparation Method:

- Cook chicken in a pan until no longer pink.
- Steam broccoli and carrots until tender.
- Serve chicken and vegetables over brown rice, drizzled with teriyaki sauce.

Calories: 400 per bowl

Lunch Recipes: Portable Lunch Ideas for Work or School

1. Mason Jar Salad

Ingredients:

- 1/4 cup balsamic vinaigrette
- 1 cup mixed greens
- 1/2 cup cherry tomatoes, halved
- 1/2 cup cucumber, diced
- 1/4 cup feta cheese, crumbled
- 1/4 cup roasted chickpeas

Preparation Method:

- Layer ingredients in a mason jar, starting with the vinaigrette at the bottom.
- Add mixed greens, then vegetables, feta cheese, and top with roasted chickpeas.
- When ready to eat, shake the jar to distribute the dressing.

Calories: 350 per jar

2. Quinoa and Black Bean Salad

Ingredients:

- 1 cup cooked quinoa
- 1/2 cup black beans, drained and rinsed
- 1/2 cup corn kernels
- 1/4 cup red bell pepper, diced
- 1/4 cup cilantro, chopped
- 2 tbsp lime juice
- Salt and pepper to taste

Preparation Method:

- Combine quinoa, black beans, corn, bell pepper, and cilantro in a bowl.
- Drizzle with lime juice and season with salt and pepper.

- Mix well and store in a portable container.

Calories: 300 per serving

These recipes are designed to provide nutritious and delicious options for lunch, catering to various dietary needs while ensuring ease of preparation and portability.

Chapter 3: Dinner Recipes

Easy One-Pan Meals

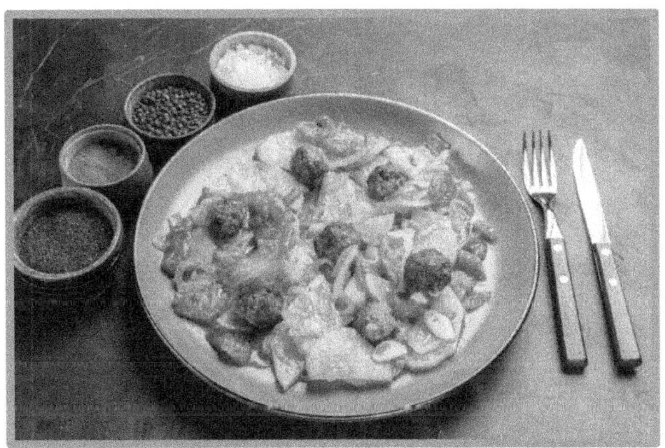

Recipe: Lemon Herb Chicken with Vegetables

Ingredients:

- 4 chicken thighs
- 1 lemon (sliced)
- 2 tbsp olive oil
- 1 tsp dried rosemary
- 1 tsp dried thyme
- 1 tsp garlic powder

- 2 cups baby potatoes (halved)
- 1 cup baby carrots
- 1 cup green beans
- Salt and pepper to taste

Preparation Method:

- Preheat your oven to 400°F (200°C).
- In a large bowl, mix the olive oil, rosemary, thyme, garlic powder, salt, and pepper.
- Add the chicken thighs to the bowl and coat them well with the seasoning mixture.
- Place the chicken thighs on a baking sheet. Arrange the baby potatoes, carrots, and green beans around the chicken.
- Top with lemon slices.
- Bake for 35-40 minutes, until the chicken is cooked through and the vegetables are tender.

Calories per Serving: 450

Flavorful Stir-Fries and Skillets

Recipe: Beef and Broccoli Stir-Fry

Ingredients:

- 1 lb beef sirloin (sliced thinly)
- 3 cups broccoli florets
- 1 bell pepper (sliced)
- 3 tbsp coconut aminos (soy sauce substitute)
- 1 tbsp sesame oil
- 2 cloves garlic (minced)
- 1 inch ginger (grated)
- 1 tbsp arrowroot starch (optional, for thickening)
- 1 tbsp water
- 2 tbsp olive oil
- Salt and pepper to taste

Preparation Method:

- In a small bowl, mix the coconut aminos, sesame oil, garlic, and ginger. Set aside.
- Heat olive oil in a large skillet over medium-high heat.
- Add the beef slices and cook until browned, about 5 minutes.
- Add the broccoli and bell pepper to the skillet. Cook for another 5 minutes, until the vegetables are tender-crisp.
- Pour the sauce over the beef and vegetables. Stir to coat everything evenly.
- If you prefer a thicker sauce, mix the arrowroot starch and water in a small bowl and add to the skillet, stirring until the sauce thickens.

Calories per Serving: 380

Slow Cooker and Instant Pot Favorites

Recipe: Slow Cooker Pulled Pork

Ingredients:

- 2 lbs pork shoulder
- 1 cup bone broth
- 1/4 cup apple cider vinegar
- 2 tbsp smoked paprika
- 1 tbsp garlic powder
- 1 tbsp onion powder
- 1 tsp black pepper
- 1 tsp sea salt

Preparation Method:

- In a small bowl, combine the smoked paprika, garlic powder, onion powder, black pepper, and salt.
- Rub the spice mixture all over the pork shoulder.
- Place the pork in the slow cooker and pour in the bone broth and apple cider vinegar.

- Cover and cook on low for 8-10 hours, or until the pork is tender and easily shredded with a fork.
- Remove the pork from the slow cooker and shred with two forks.
- Return the shredded pork to the slow cooker to soak up the juices before serving.

Calories per Serving: 350

Comforting Casseroles

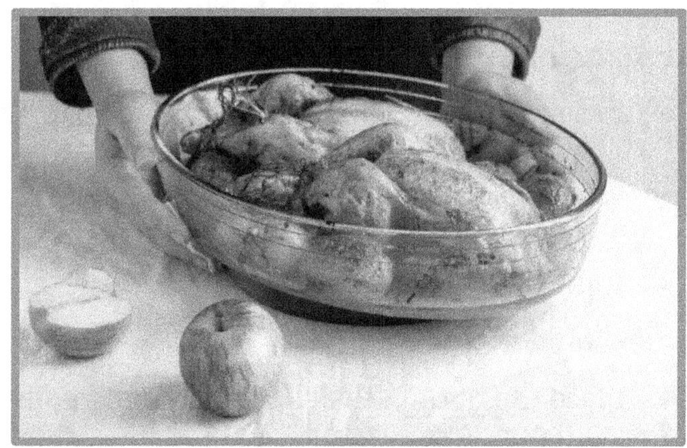

Recipe: Sweet Potato and Ground Beef Casserole

Ingredients:

- 1 lb ground beef
- 2 large sweet potatoes (peeled and sliced thinly)
- 1 onion (chopped)
- 2 cloves garlic (minced)
- 1 cup bone broth
- 1 tsp dried thyme
- 1 tsp dried oregano
- 2 tbsp olive oil
- Salt and pepper to taste

Preparation Method:

- Preheat your oven to 375°F (190°C).
- Heat olive oil in a skillet over medium heat. Add the onion and garlic, cooking until translucent.
- Add the ground beef, breaking it up with a spoon, and cook until browned.
- Stir in the thyme, oregano, salt, and pepper.

- In a baking dish, layer half of the sweet potato slices on the bottom.
- Spread the ground beef mixture over the sweet potatoes.
- Top with the remaining sweet potato slices.
- Pour the bone broth over the casserole.
- Cover with foil and bake for 45 minutes, then remove the foil and bake for an additional 15 minutes, until the sweet potatoes are tender.

Calories per Serving: 420

Seafood and Poultry Dishes

Recipe: Baked Salmon with Asparagus

Ingredients:

- 4 salmon fillets
- 1 bunch asparagus (trimmed)
- 2 tbsp olive oil
- 2 cloves garlic (minced)
- 1 lemon (sliced)

- Salt and pepper to taste
- Fresh dill for garnish

Preparation Method:
- Preheat your oven to 400°F (200°C).
- Place the salmon fillets and asparagus on a baking sheet.
- Drizzle with olive oil and sprinkle with minced garlic, salt, and pepper.
- Place lemon slices over the salmon.
- Bake for 15-20 minutes, until the salmon is cooked through and flakes easily with a fork, and the asparagus is tender.
- Garnish with fresh dill before serving.

Calories per Serving: 350

Each recipe in this section provides a flavorful and nutritious dinner option that aligns with a healthy eating plan. Enjoy the variety and simplicity of these dishes as part of a balanced diet.

Chapter 4: Snacks and Appetizers

Simple and Quick Snacks

1. Apple Slices with Coconut Butter

Ingredients:
- 1 large apple
- 2 tablespoons coconut butter

Preparation:
- Wash and core the apple.
- Slice the apple into thin wedges.
- Spread coconut butter on each apple slice.

Calories: 180 per serving

2. Carrot and Cucumber Sticks with Avocado Dip

Ingredients:

- 2 large carrots
- 1 cucumber
- 1 ripe avocado
- 1 tablespoon lemon juice
- Salt to taste

Preparation:

- Peel and cut carrots and cucumber into sticks.
- Mash the avocado in a bowl, add lemon juice and salt, and mix well.
- Serve the vegetable sticks with the avocado dip.

Calories: 150 per serving

3. Dried Fruit and Coconut Energy Balls

Ingredients:

- 1 cup pitted dates
- 1/2 cup unsweetened shredded coconut
- 1/4 cup raw pumpkin seeds

Preparation:

- Blend dates, shredded coconut, and pumpkin seeds in a food processor until well combined.
- Roll the mixture into small balls.
- Chill in the refrigerator for at least 30 minutes before serving.

Calories: 200 per serving (2 balls)

Vegetable Chips and Dips

1. Kale Chips

Ingredients:

- 1 bunch of kale
- 1 tablespoon olive oil
- Sea salt to taste

Preparation:

- Preheat oven to 350°F (175°C).

- Wash and dry the kale, remove the stems, and tear the leaves into bite-sized pieces.
- Toss the kale with olive oil and sea salt.
- Spread the kale on a baking sheet and bake for 10-15 minutes until crispy.

Calories: 50 per serving

2. Sweet Potato Chips

Ingredients:
- 2 large sweet potatoes
- 2 tablespoons olive oil
- Sea salt to taste

Preparation:
- Preheat oven to 375°F (190°C).
- Wash and thinly slice the sweet potatoes.
- Toss the slices with olive oil and sea salt.
- Arrange the slices in a single layer on a baking sheet.

- Bake for 20-25 minutes, flipping halfway through, until crispy.

Calories: 120 per serving

3. Cauliflower Hummus

Ingredients:
- 1 medium cauliflower, chopped
- 2 tablespoons tahini
- 2 tablespoons olive oil
- 2 cloves garlic
- Juice of 1 lemon
- Sea salt to taste

Preparation:
- Steam the cauliflower until tender.
- Blend the cauliflower with tahini, olive oil, garlic, lemon juice, and sea salt until smooth.
- Serve with vegetable sticks or chips.

Calories: 100 per serving

AIP-Friendly Crackers and Breads

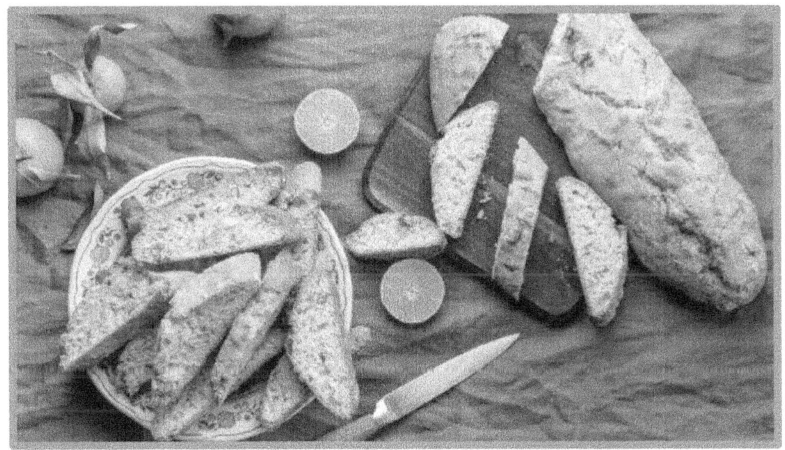

1. Plantain Crackers

Ingredients:

- 2 green plantains
- 2 tablespoons olive oil
- Sea salt to taste

Preparation:

- Preheat oven to 350°F (175°C).

- Peel and slice the plantains.
- Blend the plantains with olive oil and sea salt until smooth.
- Spread the mixture thinly on a baking sheet lined with parchment paper.
- Bake for 15-20 minutes until crispy.

Calories: 150 per serving

2. Cassava Flour Flatbread

Ingredients:

- 1 cup cassava flour
- 1/4 cup olive oil
- 1/2 cup warm water
- Sea salt to taste

Preparation:

- Mix cassava flour, olive oil, warm water, and sea salt until a dough forms.
- Divide the dough into small balls and flatten into rounds.

- Cook on a hot skillet for 2-3 minutes on each
  side until golden brown.

Calories: 180 per serving

3. Sweet Potato Biscuits

Ingredients:
- 1 cup mashed sweet potato
- 1 cup cassava flour
- 1/4 cup coconut oil, melted
- 1/2 teaspoon baking soda

Preparation:
- Preheat oven to 375°F (190°C).
- Mix all ingredients until well combined.
- Form dough into small biscuits and place on
  a baking sheet.
- Bake for 20 minutes until golden brown.

Calories: 200 per serving

Protein-Packed Bites

1. Turkey Meatballs

Ingredients:

- 1 pound ground turkey
- 1/4 cup chopped fresh parsley
- 2 cloves garlic, minced
- 1 egg (optional, if tolerated)
- Sea salt to taste

Preparation:

- Preheat oven to 375°F (190°C).
- Mix all ingredients in a bowl.
- Form mixture into small meatballs and place on a baking sheet.
- Bake for 20-25 minutes until cooked through.

Calories: 150 per serving (3 meatballs)

2. Salmon Patties

Ingredients:

- 1 can wild-caught salmon, drained
- 1/4 cup chopped green onion
- 1/4 cup cassava flour
- 1 egg (optional, if tolerated)
- 1 tablespoon coconut oil for frying

Preparation:

- Mix salmon, green onion, cassava flour, and egg in a bowl.
- Form mixture into patties.
- Heat coconut oil in a skillet over medium heat and cook patties for 3-4 minutes on each side until golden brown.

__Calories__ 180 per serving (2 patties)

3. Chicken and Spinach Mini Frittatas

Ingredients:

- 1 cup cooked chicken, shredded
- 1 cup spinach, chopped

- 6 eggs
- Sea salt to taste

Preparation:
- Preheat oven to 350°F (175°C).
- Mix all ingredients in a bowl.
- Pour mixture into a greased muffin tin.
- Bake for 20-25 minutes until set.

<u>Calories:</u> 200 per serving (2 frittatas)

Party-Ready Appetizers

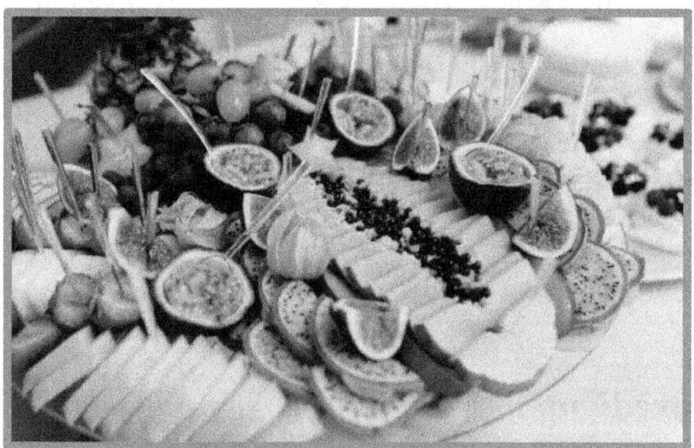

1. Bacon-Wrapped Asparagus

Ingredients:

- 1 bunch asparagus
- 8 slices of nitrate-free bacon

Preparation:

- Preheat oven to 400°F (200°C).
- Wash and trim the asparagus.
- Wrap each asparagus spear with a slice of bacon.
- Place on a baking sheet and bake for 15-20 minutes until bacon is crispy.

<u>Calories:</u> 120 per serving (2 spears)

2. Shrimp and Avocado Bites

Ingredients:

- 1 pound cooked shrimp
- 2 avocados, diced
- 1 tablespoon lemon juice
- Fresh cilantro for garnish

Preparation:

- Arrange shrimp on a platter.
- Top each shrimp with a piece of diced avocado.
- Drizzle with lemon juice and garnish with cilantro.

<u>Calories:</u> 150 per serving (4 bites)

3. Stuffed Mini Peppers

Ingredients:

- 12 mini bell peppers
- 1 cup ground turkey or beef, cooked
- 1/2 cup cauliflower rice
- 1/4 cup chopped fresh parsley
- Sea salt to taste

Preparation:

- Preheat oven to 375°F (190°C).

- Cut the tops off the mini peppers and remove seeds.
- Mix cooked ground meat, cauliflower rice, parsley, and sea salt.
- Stuff the peppers with the meat mixture.
- Place on a baking sheet and bake for 15-20 minutes until peppers are tender.

Calories: 180 per serving (3 peppers)

Chapter 5: Desserts and Treats

Naturally Sweetened Delights

Desserts are often seen as indulgences, but when naturally sweetened and aligned with the principles of an autoimmune protocol (AIP) diet, they can be both delicious and beneficial to health. Naturally sweetened delights focus on using ingredients like fruits, honey, and maple syrup, which provide sweetness without the negative impact of refined sugars.

Recipes:

1. **Banana Coconut Ice Cream**
2. **Honey-Sweetened Apple Crisp**
3. **Maple Pecan Bites**

1. Banana Coconut Ice Cream

Ingredients:

- 4 ripe bananas
- 1 can of full-fat coconut milk
- 1 teaspoon vanilla extract

Preparation Method:

- Slice the bananas and freeze them for at least 2 hours or overnight.
- In a food processor, blend the frozen banana slices until smooth.
- Add the coconut milk and vanilla extract, and blend until well combined.
- Pour the mixture into an ice cream maker and churn according to the manufacturer's instructions. Alternatively, pour into a freezer-safe container and freeze for 2-3 hours, stirring every 30 minutes to break up ice crystals.
- Serve immediately or store in the freezer for later.

<u>***Calories per Serving (1/2 cup):***</u> Approximately 120 calories

2. Honey-Sweetened Apple Crisp

Ingredients:
- 4 medium apples, peeled and sliced
- 1/4 cup honey
- 1 teaspoon cinnamon
- 1/2 cup coconut flour
- 1/2 cup shredded coconut
- 1/4 cup coconut oil, melted

Preparation Method:
- Preheat the oven to 350°F (175°C).
- In a mixing bowl, combine the apple slices, honey, and cinnamon. Toss to coat the apples evenly.
- Transfer the apple mixture to a baking dish.

- In another bowl, mix the coconut flour, shredded coconut, and melted coconut oil until crumbly.
- Sprinkle the coconut mixture over the apples.
- Bake for 30-35 minutes, or until the topping is golden brown and the apples are tender.
- Allow to cool slightly before serving.

Calories per Serving (1/6 of recipe):

Approximately 220 calories

3. Maple Pecan Bites

Ingredients:

- 1 cup pecans
- 1/4 cup almond flour
- 2 tablespoons maple syrup
- 1 teaspoon vanilla extract
- A pinch of sea salt

Preparation Method:

- Preheat the oven to 350°F (175°C).

- In a food processor, pulse the pecans until they are finely chopped.
- In a bowl, combine the chopped pecans, almond flour, maple syrup, vanilla extract, and sea salt. Mix until well combined.
- Roll the mixture into small balls and place them on a parchment-lined baking sheet.
- Bake for 10-12 minutes, or until the bites are golden brown.
- Allow to cool completely before serving.

Calories per Bite (makes 12): Approximately 80 calories

Grain-Free Cookies and Bars

For those following an AIP diet, grain-free cookies and bars offer a satisfying alternative to traditional baked goods. These treats are crafted to avoid common allergens and inflammatory ingredients, using nutrient-dense components that align with the AIP principles.

1. Coconut Flour Chocolate Chip Cookies

2. Pumpkin Spice Bars

3. Lemon Coconut Bars

1. Coconut Flour Chocolate Chip Cookies

Ingredients:

- 1/2 cup coconut flour
- 1/4 cup coconut oil, melted
- 1/4 cup honey
- 2 large eggs
- 1 teaspoon vanilla extract
- 1/4 teaspoon baking soda
- 1/4 cup carob chips (AIP-friendly chocolate substitute)

Preparation Method:

- Preheat the oven to 350°F (175°C) and line a baking sheet with parchment paper.

- In a mixing bowl, whisk together the melted coconut oil, honey, eggs, and vanilla extract.
- Add the coconut flour and baking soda to the wet ingredients and mix until a dough forms.
- Fold in the carob chips.
- Drop tablespoon-sized portions of dough onto the prepared baking sheet, flattening each slightly with the back of a spoon.
- Bake for 10-12 minutes, or until the edges are golden brown.
- Allow to cool on the baking sheet for a few minutes before transferring to a wire rack to cool completely.

Calories per Cookie (makes 12): Approximately 120 calories

2. Pumpkin Spice Bars

Ingredients:
- 1 cup pumpkin puree
- 1/2 cup coconut flour

- 1/4 cup maple syrup
- 2 large eggs
- 1/4 cup coconut oil, melted
- 1 teaspoon cinnamon
- 1/2 teaspoon nutmeg
- 1/2 teaspoon baking soda
- A/ pinch of sea salt

Preparation Method:

- Preheat the oven to 350°F (175°C) and line an 8x8-inch baking dish with parchment paper.
- In a large bowl, mix together the pumpkin puree, maple syrup, eggs, and melted coconut oil.
- In a separate bowl, whisk together the coconut flour, cinnamon, nutmeg, baking soda, and sea salt.
- Gradually add the dry ingredients to the wet ingredients, stirring until well combined.
- Pour the batter into the prepared baking dish and spread evenly.

- Bake for 25-30 minutes, or until a toothpick inserted into the center comes out clean.
- Allow to cool completely before cutting into bars.

Calories per Bar (makes 9): Approximately 150 calories

3. Lemon Coconut Bars

Ingredients:
- 1/2 cup coconut flour
- 1/4 cup coconut oil, melted
- 1/4 cup honey
- 2 large eggs
- Zest and juice of 2 lemons
- 1/2 teaspoon vanilla extract

Preparation Method:
- Preheat the oven to 350°F (175°C) and line an 8x8-inch baking dish with parchment paper.

- In a mixing bowl, combine the melted coconut oil, honey, eggs, lemon zest, lemon juice, and vanilla extract.
- Add the coconut flour to the wet ingredients and mix until a thick batter forms.
- Pour the batter into the prepared baking dish and spread evenly.
- Bake for 20-25 minutes, or until the edges are golden brown and the center is set.
- Allow to cool completely before cutting into bars.

Calories per Bar (makes 9): Approximately 130 calories

These naturally sweetened and grain-free treats offer satisfying and health-conscious alternatives to traditional desserts, making them perfect for anyone following an AIP diet. They are not only delicious but also designed to help manage autoimmune symptoms by avoiding common triggers and focusing on nutrient-dense ingredients.

Refreshing Frozen Treats

When managing an autoimmune condition, finding satisfying and compliant frozen treats can be a challenge. The key is to create delicious, refreshing desserts that align with the principles of the Autoimmune Protocol (AIP) diet. Below are some delightful recipes that will help you beat the heat while staying on track with your dietary needs.

Coconut Mango Popsicles

Ingredients:

- 2 cups fresh or frozen mango chunks
- 1 can (13.5 oz) full-fat coconut milk
- 2 tablespoons honey (optional, adjust based on sweetness of mangoes)
- 1 teaspoon vanilla extract (AIP-compliant)

Preparation Method:

- In a blender, combine the mango chunks,
  coconut milk, honey, and vanilla extract.
- Blend until smooth and creamy.
- Pour the mixture into popsicle molds, leaving
  a little space at the top for expansion.
- Insert popsicle sticks and freeze for at least 4
  hours, or until solid.
- To release the popsicles from the molds, run
  warm water over the outside of the molds for
  a few seconds.

Calories: Approximately 130 calories per popsicle

Blueberry Coconut Ice Cream

Ingredients:
- 2 cups fresh or frozen blueberries
- 1 can (13.5 oz) full-fat coconut milk
- 3 tablespoons honey
- 1 tablespoon lemon juice

Preparation Method:

- In a medium saucepan, combine blueberries, honey, and lemon juice. Cook over medium heat until the blueberries start to burst and release their juices, about 5-7 minutes.
- Remove from heat and let cool slightly.
- In a blender, combine the blueberry mixture and coconut milk. Blend until smooth.
- Pour the mixture into an ice cream maker and churn according to the manufacturer's instructions.
- Transfer the ice cream to a freezer-safe container and freeze for at least 2 hours before serving.

Calories: Approximately 160 calories per serving

Strawberry Banana Sorbet

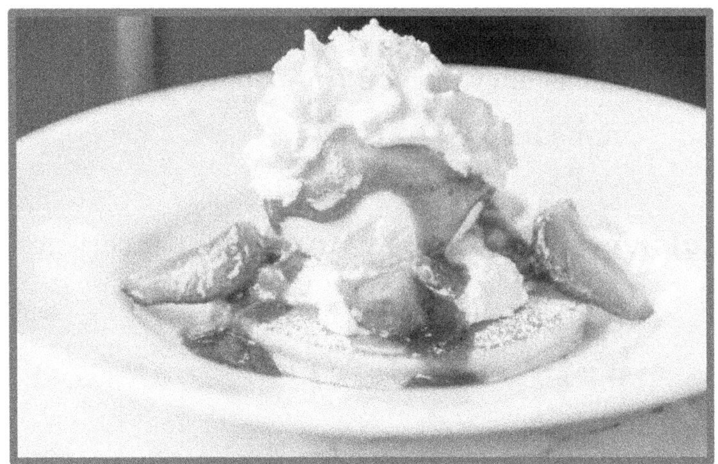

Ingredients:

- 2 cups fresh or frozen strawberries
- 1 ripe banana
- 2 tablespoons honey
- 1 teaspoon lemon juice

Preparation Method:

- In a blender, combine strawberries, banana, honey, and lemon juice.
- Blend until smooth and creamy.
- Pour the mixture into a shallow dish and freeze for about 2 hours, stirring every 30 minutes to break up ice crystals.

- Once the sorbet has reached the desired consistency, scoop into bowls and serve immediately.

<u>Calories:</u> Approximately 110 calories per serving

Holiday and Special Occasion Sweets

Celebrating holidays and special occasions can be challenging when following the AIP diet, but it's entirely possible to create delicious and festive sweets that comply with the dietary guidelines. Here are some AIP-friendly recipes to help you enjoy those special moments without compromising your health.

Gingerbread Cookies

Ingredients:
- 1 cup coconut flour

- 1/2 cup tapioca flour
- 1/2 cup molasses
- 1/4 cup coconut oil, melted
- 1 teaspoon ground ginger
- 1 teaspoon ground cinnamon
- 1/4 teaspoon ground cloves
- 1/4 teaspoon sea salt

Preparation Method:

- Preheat the oven to 350°F (175°C) and line a baking sheet with parchment paper.
- In a large bowl, mix together the coconut flour, tapioca flour, ginger, cinnamon, cloves, and sea salt.
- Add the molasses and melted coconut oil to the dry ingredients and stir until well combined. The dough should be thick and pliable.
- Roll the dough into small balls and flatten them slightly onto the prepared baking sheet.
- Bake for 10-12 minutes, or until the edges are golden brown.

- Let the cookies cool on the baking sheet for a few minutes before transferring them to a wire rack to cool completely.

<u>Calories:</u> Approximately 80 calories per cookie

Apple Cinnamon Crumble

Ingredients:
- 4 large apples, peeled, cored, and sliced
- 1/4 cup honey
- 1 tablespoon lemon juice
- 1 teaspoon ground cinnamon
- 1/2 cup coconut flour
- 1/4 cup coconut oil, melted
- 1/4 cup shredded coconut

Preparation Method:
- Preheat the oven to 350°F (175°C).
- In a large bowl, combine the apple slices, honey, lemon juice, and cinnamon. Toss to coat the apples evenly.

- Transfer the apple mixture to a baking dish.
- In a separate bowl, mix together the coconut flour, melted coconut oil, and shredded coconut until crumbly.
- Sprinkle the crumble mixture evenly over the apples.
- Bake for 25-30 minutes, or until the apples are tender and the crumble topping is golden brown.
- Let cool slightly before serving.

Calories: Approximately 190 calories per serving

Pumpkin Pie Bars

Ingredients:
- 1 cup pumpkin puree
- 1/2 cup coconut milk
- 1/4 cup honey
- 2 tablespoons coconut flour
- 1 teaspoon ground cinnamon
- 1/2 teaspoon ground ginger

- 1/4 teaspoon ground nutmeg
- 1/4 teaspoon sea salt

Preparation Method:

- Preheat the oven to 350°F (175°C) and line an 8x8-inch baking dish with parchment paper.
- In a large bowl, combine the pumpkin puree, coconut milk, honey, coconut flour, cinnamon, ginger, nutmeg, and sea salt. Mix until smooth.
- Pour the mixture into the prepared baking dish and spread evenly.
- Bake for 25-30 minutes, or until the center is set and the edges are lightly browned.
- Let cool completely before cutting into bars.

Calories: Approximately 140 calories per bar

These recipes offer a variety of flavors and textures to keep your taste buds delighted while staying compliant with the AIP diet. Whether you're enjoying a refreshing frozen treat on a hot day or celebrating a special occasion, these recipes ensure you can indulge without compromising your health.

Conclusion

Embarking on the journey of managing autoimmune diseases through dietary changes can be both challenging and rewarding. The Autoimmune Protocol (AIP) diet, as presented in "The Complete Autoimmune Cookbook for Beginners," offers a structured yet flexible approach to help individuals reduce inflammation, support gut health, and improve their overall well-being. As we conclude this comprehensive guide, it is important to reflect on the principles, practices, and personal growth that come with embracing the AIP diet.

The AIP diet is not merely a temporary dietary adjustment; it is a holistic lifestyle change that emphasizes the importance of nutrient-dense foods, mindful eating, and self-awareness. By eliminating potential dietary triggers and focusing on whole, unprocessed foods, the AIP diet aims to calm the immune system and promote healing. This approach requires patience, dedication, and a willingness to listen to your body's unique needs.

One of the most significant aspects of the AIP diet is its personalization. Each individual's experience with autoimmune diseases and dietary responses is unique. The elimination phase of the AIP diet serves as a powerful tool to identify specific food sensitivities and triggers. By systematically reintroducing foods, you can tailor the diet to meet your personal needs, ensuring that you are nourishing your body in the best possible way. This process of discovery fosters a deeper understanding of your body's signals and how various foods affect your health.

Incorporating a variety of nutrient-dense foods is a cornerstone of the AIP diet. The focus on fruits, vegetables, high-quality proteins, and healthy fats ensures that your diet is balanced and provides essential vitamins and minerals. These nutrients play crucial roles in supporting immune function, reducing inflammation, and enhancing overall health. By embracing this diverse range of foods, you not only improve your nutritional intake but also enjoy a rich tapestry of flavors and textures that make the diet enjoyable and sustainable.

Adopting the AIP diet also encourages a mindful and intentional approach to eating. Preparing meals from scratch, experimenting with new ingredients, and savoring the flavors of wholesome foods can transform your relationship with food. This mindful eating practice promotes a greater appreciation for the nourishment that food provides and reinforces the connection between diet and health. It can also be a source of joy and creativity, turning meal preparation into a rewarding experience.

While the AIP diet offers numerous benefits, it is important to recognize that the journey may come with challenges. Social situations, holidays, and special occasions can pose difficulties, but with planning and creativity, you can navigate these events while staying true to your dietary goals. The recipes and tips provided in this cookbook are designed to help you enjoy these moments without compromising your health. Learning to adapt and find balance in various contexts is key to long-term success.

Support and community are invaluable resources on this journey. Connecting with others who share your experiences can provide encouragement, practical tips, and a sense of camaraderie. Whether through support groups, online communities, or social media platforms, these connections can make the journey less isolating and more manageable. Additionally, collaborating with healthcare professionals who are knowledgeable about the AIP diet and autoimmune diseases can provide personalized guidance and support, ensuring that your dietary changes are safe and effective.

In conclusion, the AIP diet represents a comprehensive approach to managing autoimmune diseases through informed dietary choices and lifestyle changes. By following the principles outlined in this cookbook, you are taking proactive steps towards improving your health and well-being. The journey may require effort and adjustment, but the potential rewards—reduced inflammation, improved symptoms, and enhanced quality of life—make it worthwhile.

Remember, the AIP diet is a tool for empowerment. It equips you with the knowledge and resources to make informed decisions about your health. As you continue on this path, stay curious, stay flexible, and stay committed to your well-being. Celebrate your successes, learn from your challenges, and take pride in the strides you are making towards better health.

"The Complete Autoimmune Cookbook for Beginners" is more than just a collection of recipes; it is a guide and companion in your journey to healing. May it serve as a source of inspiration, comfort, and empowerment as you navigate the complexities of autoimmune health. Your commitment to this journey is a testament to your dedication to living a healthier, more vibrant life. Here's to your continued success and well-being.